"I AM THE LO
IS THERE AN
—JEREMIAH 32:27

A STUDY GUIDE FOR
TRUSTING *God* with CANCER

ROB RABAN
Author and Cancer Survivor

With Lisa Guest

A Study Guide for Trusting God with Cancer
Copyright © 2020 by Rob Raban

All rights reserved.

Published in the United States by Rob Raban LLC.

Edited by Lisa Guest

Formatting by Christian Editing Services (www.christianeditingservices.com)

No portion of this book may be reproduced, stored in a retrieval system, or transmitted in any form or by any means—electronic, mechanical, photocopy, recording, scanning, or other—except for brief quotations in critical reviews or articles, without the prior written permission of the publisher.

Unless otherwise indicated, Scripture quotations are taken from *The Holy Bible, New International Version*®, **NIV® Copyright © 1973, 1978, 1984, 2011 by Biblica, Inc.® Used by permission. All rights reserved worldwide.**

Scripture quotations marked ESV are from *The English Standard Version.* © 2001 by Crossway Bibles, a division of Good News Publishers. Used by permission.

Scripture quotations marked NLT are from *Holy Bible, New Living Translation.* © 1996, 2004, 2007, 2013. Used by permission of Tyndale House Publishers, Inc., Carol Stream, Ill. 60188. All rights reserved.

Scripture quotations marked NKJV are from *The New King James Version.* © 1982 by Thomas Nelson, Inc. Used by permission. All rights reserved.

LIBRARY OF CONGRESS CATALOGUING-IN-PUBLICATION DATA

Raban, Rob.

Trusting God with Cancer / Rob Raban

Table of Contents

A Word to Leaders	5
Foreword	9
Lesson 1. Misdiagnosing a Sneeze	13
Lesson 2. "Your Cancer Is Doubling on the Hour"	18
Lesson 3. Finding New Hope	22
Lesson 4. Telling the Kids	29
Lesson 5. Dreams That Matter	37
Lesson 6. A Week of Testing	42
Lesson 7. "Have a *Little* Faith"	51
Lesson 8. Chemo: Embrace It!	57
Lesson 9. Family, Friends, and the Internet	66
Lesson 10. Signs and Miracles	74
Lesson 11. Strategies to Beat Cancer	80
Epilogue	87
Resources	93
The First Step: An Invitation	93
A Handful of Foundation Truths About God	94
Finding Answers to Questions	94
Ideas for Leaders: Opening Each Group Time	95

A Word to Leaders

First—before we get to business matters—thank you for stepping forward. You may not truly understand the importance of your role in giving people the opportunity to not be alone in their battle against cancer or in their effort to support a warrior they love. The people in your group may struggle to express their appreciation, but I can assure you that what you are doing is good and life-giving.

Also, remember that the chief value of this group is the participants' sharing in each other's personal stories. That means you, as the leader, don't have to have all the answers. So relax, take a deep breath, and trust God to equip you for the exciting journey ahead!

Now to some business items:

- The first lesson includes a kick-off welcome that can be a stand-alone or be done in conjunction with Chapter #1.

- As you familiarize yourself with the material, determine whether you want to tackle one lesson a week or two lessons a week.

- Whether you do one or two lessons a week, begin every meeting with everyone together. Share a story or question that sets up the discussion to come. At the back of the book, you'll find "Ideas for Leaders: Opening Each Group Time." As you get to know the group, though, you may want to go in different directions—and do so!

- After the large-group opening, split into two groups: CANCER FIGHTERS and CAREGIVERS. Depending on the amount of time available, choose one question from each of the three sections to focus on. You—or a co-leader who has perhaps fought cancer—will lead the CANCER FIGHTERS. If you're the only leader, take the CANCER FIGHTERS and, before the first meeting, choose a capable CAREGIVER to facilitate that discussion.

- When you have about thirty minutes remaining, come back into a large group to discuss a single question from the lesson. (In each lesson, the **asterisked question is simply a suggestion.) Ideally, during this time, CANCER FIGHTERS can learn from CAREGIVERS and CAREGIVERS, from CANCER FIGHTERS.

- In the back of the book is an invitation for participants to put their faith in Jesus as well as a list of some resources. That list is occasionally referred to in the lessons. Again, you may have some additional suggestions for your group. Don't hesitate to share those.

- Having gathered as a single group or before people leave their small group, spend some time in prayer.

  If people are comfortable praying for themselves, invite them to do so. Then you or another member of the group could pray that same request aloud.

  Another approach would be letting individuals

A Word to Leaders

share their prayer requests, and after all have shared, the group prays so that every person with a request hears himself/herself being prayed for.

Depending on the group, you may simply close the session in prayer, being sure to cover whatever specifics have been mentioned in the earlier discussion.

And you don't have to do the same thing each week.

- Close with a blessing (see Numbers 6:24-26 below) and/or a prayer, whatever is comfortable for you.

- If you want to close your study of *Trusting God with Cancer* with something social, save the epilogue for that meeting time. Another option is to do the eleventh lesson and the epilogue together at a single meeting.

- Please familiarize yourself with the resources at the back of the book: "The First Step: An Invitation" guides people to give their life to Jesus; "A Handful of Foundational Truths" is a list of some basic Scriptures about salvation; "Finding Answers to Questions" offers resources for general questions as well as some specific issues raised by several chapters; and—as mentioned above and specifically for you—"Ideas for Leaders: Opening Each Lesson."

Finally, may the Lord guide you, and may He bless you as He uses you to bless others.

Rob

*"The LORD bless you
and keep you;
the LORD make his face shine on you
and be gracious to you;
the LORD turn his face toward you
and give you peace."*

Numbers 6:24-26

Foreword

Welcome. [Briefly introduce yourself… and why you have chosen to lead this group.] Open with prayer:

> *Lord God, it is no accident that each of us is gathered here. You have called each one of us to be part of this group. May that truth make us excited about what You have for each one of us. May we read every chapter and attend every meeting with genuine anticipation of what You have for us individually. God, You know that life on this earth is hard. We call out to You for physical healing from cancer. After all, we know that You are the Lord, the God of all flesh, and that nothing is too hard for You. We believe; help our unbelief…. And please guide our conversation this next hour.*

Ask the participants to introduce themselves and, in a sentence or two, say why they joined this group.

Too many people skip a book's foreword and introduction. That's one reason why I'm going to read this foreword out loud. Another reason is, hearing these words as you read along will increase the impact of this powerful truth and the passionate encouragement of Rob Raban, whom you'll come to know well in the next several weeks. (Read "Foreword.")

There's no test, but I'd love to hear from a few of you what impacted you the most in the words I just read.

- Rob's book is called *Trusting God with Cancer*. What is the biggest thing—other than cancer—that you have ever trusted to God?

- What do (did) you do to strengthen your faith in God as you trust(ed) Him?

Thanks all of you for sharing. It's time for some housekeeping. We'll be meeting twelve more times, discussing one chapter each week. Our last meeting will be a brief discussion of the epilogue and a closing celebration.* Each chapter has three questions for you if you are battling cancer now and three questions if you are a caregiver, family member, or friend of someone dealing with cancer. We will also spend some time praying together. Ideally, each of us will be prayed for each week by someone in this circle. Hearing yourself being prayed for—and being able to feel God's love through that prayer and to piggyback on that person's faith—can be a life-giving blessing. My prayer is that this group will be safe, that you will find support from people who are walking a journey similar to yours, and that God will use our time together to grow your faith in Him.

Before our next meeting, please read chapter 1—"Misdiagnosing a Sneeze"—and answer the questions so you'll be ready to be part of the discussion.

One more thing—and I won't do this again unless you want me to. This week let's memorize Jeremiah 32:27. "I am the Lord, the God of all flesh. Is there anything too hard for Me?" The verse is printed on the front cover of your book. May its truth be a solid lifeline for you.

Close in prayer.

Forward

Finally, let me bless you with words that echo Rob's:

As you go through *Trusting God with Cancer*, may you experience the love of God and the love of His Son, Jesus Christ. May you learn to see everyday miracles in your life... and may you become more aware of the Lord's presence with you always. And whatever you're feeling—doubt, fear, anger, suspicion, lack of forgiveness, self-pity, selfishness—may God move those mountains out of your life.

* Another option: We'll be meeting six more times, discussing two chapters each week.

Lesson 1
Misdiagnosing a Sneeze

CANCER FIGHTERS

1. *"You've cracked a rib."*... *"Change deodorants."*... *"You're tired because you're a busy dad."*... *"We've found something."* Using short statements like these, talk about the steps involved until you got to the *"We've found something"* point.

2. A missed diagnosis is definitely a reason for anger—and definitely an opportunity to extend forgiveness. As author and professor Lewis Smedes put it, "To forgive is to set a prisoner free and discover that the prisoner was you."

   What forgiveness, if any, do you need to extend to someone you encountered in the medical world?

   _____

   _____

   Why are you struggling to forgive? Know that forgiving doesn't mean you approve of what the person did. It doesn't mean that a wrong wasn't done or that you're excusing the act. And forgiveness doesn't mean you suddenly trust the person or you re-enter the relationship.

_____

_____

** Why would it be good for you to forgive?

_____

_____

3. More may be involved in extending forgiveness than just forgiving people in the medical community.

Do you need to forgive yourself for anything? Maybe looking back you wish you had been more assertive with a doctor, a nurse, or even a receptionist. Be gentle with yourself: we don't know what we don't know when we're walking through a new experience.

_____

Do you need to forgive God? This heretical-sounding question is one you may wrestle with for quite a while. Know that God can handle your anger, your rage, your disappointment in Him. Don't hold back.

_____

_____

_____

Lesson 1: Misdiagnosing a Sneeze

CAREGIVERS

1. Think about the pre-diagnosis time.

   Looking back, where do you see God guiding?

   _____

   _____

   What evidence of His grace in your loved one's life
   do you see? At some point your loved one might be
   encouraged to hear your thoughts.

   _____

   _____

   _____

2. A missed diagnosis is definitely a reason for anger—and
   definitely an opportunity to extend forgiveness. As author
   and professor Lewis Smedes put it, "To forgive is to set a
   prisoner free and discover that the prisoner was you."

   What forgiveness, if any, do you need to extend
   to someone whom your loved one—or you as an
   advocate—encountered in the medical world?

   _____

   _____

   Why are you struggling to forgive? Know that forgiving
   does not mean you approve of what the person did.

Trusting God With Cancer

It doesn't mean that a wrong wasn't done or that you're excusing the act. And forgiveness doesn't mean you suddenly trust the person or you re-enter the relationship.

_____

_____

** Why would it be good for you to be able to forgive?

_____

_____

3. More may be involved in extending forgiveness than just forgiving people in the medical community.

Do you need to forgive yourself for anything? Maybe looking back you wish you had been more assertive with a doctor or nurse or even receptionist. Be gentle with yourself: we don't know what we don't know when we're walking through a new experience.

_____

_____

Do you need to forgive God? This heretical-sounding question is one you may wrestle with for quite a while. Know that God can handle your anger, your rage, your disappointment in Him. Don't hold back.

_____

Lesson 1: Misdiagnosing a Sneeze

———————————————————

———————————————————

———————————————————

*"I am the L\ORD, the God of all flesh.
Is there anything too hard for me?"*

Jeremiah 32:27

Lesson 2
"Your Cancer Is Doubling on the Hour"

CANCER FIGHTERS

1. Arms stretched out over his head and braced for the first staple-gun shot of his four-shot bone marrow biopsy, Rob suddenly had two hands holding his: Virginia, his nurse, helped Rob "stare down a room full of steel and uncertainty... and feel secure."

    Who was/is a Virginia in your journey?

    _____

    In what other ways did God—early on—make it clear to you that He would comfort you and protect you, that you would not fight this battle alone? Your initial answer might be a reflexive "God wasn't there." But take a moment to look back—maybe ask God to show you—and you just may see His presence in retrospect when you didn't notice it in real time. (We all do that!)

Lesson 2: "Your Cancer is Doubling on the Hour"

_____

_____

_____

_____

2. Barbi, Rob's wife, was a bold and persistent advocate, tracking down test results, addressing incompetent office staff, and calling out inept doctors. Also, at the initial oncologist appointment, Rob and Barbi were joined by their friend Karen who had been an oncology nurse before choosing to be at home with her children.

    Think about the people God has put in your life for this fight. Which one or two seemed truly sent by God to battle with you and for you?

    _____

3. Hearing the diagnosis and feeling Barbi's trembling arm, Rob stood to his feet and—uncharacteristically—prayed boldly: Rob acknowledged God's sovereignty and healing power.

    ** We all go through seasons when prayer comes fairly easily and those when we find ourselves hardly praying at all. What impact has your diagnosis had on your prayer life?

    _____

Trusting God With Cancer

_____

_____

Understandably your faith may have been and may still be something of a roller coaster ride. What impact has your diagnosis had on your faith overall? If you are wrestling with why God allows bad things to happen, take a look at page 93 for resources.

_____

_____

CAREGIVERS

1. It's hard to helplessly watch someone you love go through a difficult time. In what ways could you be a Virginia for your loved one? Be specific. Brainstorm with other members of this group.

_____

_____

_____

2. Some people are advocates, others are medical professionals, and still others have survived cancer themselves. Some people are natural encouragers, others are gifted in prayer, and still others know just the right Scripture verse to turn to. Each person brings experience

Lesson 2: "Your Cancer is Doubling on the Hour"

and/or knowledge to the life of a CANCER FIGHTER.

What role in your loved one's life has God called you to?

_____

In what ways have you experienced God's presence and/or His empowerment?

_____

_____

_____

3. We all go through seasons when prayer comes fairly easily and those when we find ourselves hardly praying at all.

    ** What impact has your loved one's diagnosis had on your prayer life?

    _____

    _____

    Understandably your faith may have been something of a roller coaster ride. What impact has your loved one's diagnosis had on your faith overall? If you are wrestling with why God allows bad things to happen, take a look at page 93 for resources.

    The LORD is my strength and my shield;
    My heart trusts in him, and he helps me.

    Psalm 28:7

Lesson 3
Finding New Hope

CANCER FIGHTERS

1. Review—and, when you're in your group, read aloud—what Rob says on pages 27-28. Then, for a few minutes, think about what you think about.

    Which of your regular thoughts are healing thoughts? If you have none or only a few, find some more (maybe from people in this group). What will you do to stay focused on those healing thoughts?

    _____

    _____

    Which of your regular thoughts are *not* healing thoughts? What could you do to minimize the time you spend with them?

    _____

    _____

Lesson 3: Finding New Hope

2. Compare and contrast your experience to Rob's.

In what ways has a diagnosis of cancer clarified your thoughts and rearranged priorities? Be specific.

_____

_____

_____

_____

Think about the grief and pain you felt when you first heard the diagnosis. What, if anything, gave you relief? What do you do for yourself these days when you feel discouraged and/or when the grief overwhelms?

_____

_____

_____

_____

When, if ever, have your tears been purifying? If you haven't experienced this, consider in what ways tears might be purifying.

_____

_____

_____

Trusting God With Cancer

What factors contributed to your choice of oncologist? What evidence do you see of God's role in your finding that doctor?

———————————————————————————

———————————————————————————

———————————————————————————

3. Rob is very open about the fact that God is integral to the process of raging, grieving, and accepting: "Whether or not you believe in Him, if you've been diagnosed with a life-threatening disease, your fears and your anger will sooner or later lead you to a direct confrontation with God. Specifically, you will have to wrestle with whether God is truly an all-knowing, all-powerful, all-loving God... or not" (page 33). On page 36, Rob shares a little about his faith in God.

Describe any confrontation you've had with God... before cancer as well as since the diagnosis.

———————————————————————————

———————————————————————————

———————————————————————————

———————————————————————————

———————————————————————————

———————————————————————————

Lesson 3: Finding New Hope

** If you're already relying on God as you battle this evil disease, share with the group the value of your relationship with Jesus at this time.

If you're skeptical about God, that's absolutely OK. He can handle our skepticism as well as our anger. Someone in the group may be a good person to talk to if you have questions—even hard questions—about God. If you'd like answers to those questions, take a look at page 93 for resources.

CAREGIVERS

1. On pages 27-28, Rob talks about thoughts that would heal him and those that wouldn't. Similarly, as a CAREGIVER, you can choose to focus on thoughts that are helpful and those that are not.

    Which of your regular thoughts are helpful? If you have none or only a few, find some more (maybe from people in this group). What will you do to stay focused on these helpful thoughts?

    _____

    _____

    _____

    _____

    _____

Trusting God With Cancer

Which of your regular thoughts are *not* helpful? What will you do to minimize the time you spend with them?

_____

_____

_____

_____

_____

2. Since Rob writes from the perspective of a CANCER FIGHTER, you as a CAREGIVER can gain insight into the thoughts and emotions your loved one may be experiencing.

In what ways has your loved one's diagnosis of cancer clarified your thoughts and rearranged your priorities? Be specific.

_____

_____

_____

_____

_____

Describe the grief and pain you felt when you first heard your loved one's diagnosis. What at the time, if anything, gave you relief? What do you do for yourself

Lesson 3: Finding New Hope

when you feel discouraged and/or when the grief overwhelms?

_____

_____

_____

When, if ever, have your tears been purifying? If you haven't experienced it, consider in what ways tears might be purifying.

_____

_____

What evidence do you see of God's role in your loved one finding his/her oncologist?

_____

_____

3. Rob is very open about the fact that God is integral to the process of raging, grieving, and accepting: "Whether or not you believe in Him, if you've been diagnosed with a life-threatening disease, your fears and your anger will sooner or later lead you to a direct confrontation with God. Specifically, you will have to wrestle with whether God is truly an all-knowing, all-powerful, all-loving God… or not" (page 33). On page 36, Rob shares a little about his faith in God.

Trusting God With Cancer

Describe your relationship with God... before your loved one's diagnosis and after.

_____

_____

_____

_____

_____

** If you were a believer before the diagnosis, share with the group the value of your relationship with Jesus during this time.

If you're skeptical about God, that's absolutely OK. He can handle our skepticism as well as our anger. Someone in the group may be a good person to talk to if you have questions—even hard questions—about God. If you'd like answers to those questions, take a look at page 93 for resources.

"Do not fear, for I am with you; do not be dismayed, for I am your God. I will strengthen you and help you. I will uphold you with my righteous right hand."

Isaiah 41:10

Lesson 4
Telling the Kids

CANCER FIGHTERS

1. A rather mild-mannered guy, not particularly bold or self-confident, Rob found that cancer unleashed a lion from within.

    What was your initial reaction to your diagnosis? Like Rob, did you find—to some degree—new strength, or boldness, or self-confidence? Or perhaps your very understandable response was terror and numbness? Maybe you accepted the diagnosis as a death sentence. What is your attitude toward the enemy and/or the battle right now? If your attitude has improved, what caused the change—and what might you do to maintain that improvement?

    _____
    _____
    _____
    _____

Trusting God With Cancer

> ** Rob recognized right away one blessing of cancer: it quickly drove him to his knees to ask for God's help. At the same time, though, cancer had Rob on his feet crying out, "This cancer is not bigger than God!" What rallying cry do you have—or might you adopt—for your battle?

_____

_____

2. When it came time to tell their kids about the cancer, Rob and Barbi chose this strategy: *Be honest with the children and invite them into the process.* Rob acknowledges that the severity of his cancer would have impacted the kind of conversation he and Barbi would have had with his sons.

   In what way(s) did you benefit from telling your children, or other family members, or close friends about your cancer diagnosis?

   _____

   _____

   What was the most helpful response? Describe that person's words and/or actions.

   _____

   _____

   People die from cancer, and addressing death is rarely easy. Briefly describe your attitude toward death and

Lesson 4: Telling the Kids

how it is impacting—positively and/or negatively—your fight. If your perspective on death is not helping, where will you turn for counsel and encouragement? If you would like to know more about death, take a look at page 93 for resources.

_____

_____

3. After watching Rob in the pool with the boys, throwing them into the air and having them splash down into the water again and again, Barbi dubbed this Raban approach to healing "the new face of cancer."

In your own personal way, what new face are you giving cancer—or would you like to give cancer? Think boldly and be specific.

_____

_____

For Rob, his physical activity and playing sports with his sons were signs of normalcy and, he noted, reassurance to the boys and to Rob himself that he was still alive. What activity, hobby, passion, or pastime might you continue with that will serve as a comforting sign of normalcy?

_____

_____

If you are a follower of Jesus, cancer is a chance to show your family—and yourself—the true meaning of faith. The diagnosis of cancer and its subsequent treatment are opportunities to demonstrate trusting your heavenly Father, praying, submitting to God's will, and asking for His help. As you battle this evil disease, what sort of example will you be for your children and anyone else who are watching you?

_____

_____

_____

CAREGIVERS

1. A rather mild-mannered guy, not particularly bold or self-confident, Rob found that cancer unleashed a lion from within. Your personality and your diagnosis were undoubtedly key factors in your response to your loved one's diagnosis.

   What was your initial reaction to the diagnosis? Like Rob, did you find—to some degree—new strength or boldness? Or perhaps your very understandable response was terror and numbness? Maybe you accepted the diagnosis as a death sentence for your loved one. What is your attitude toward the enemy and/ or the battle right now? If your attitude has improved,

Lesson 4: Telling the Kids

what caused the change—and what might you do to maintain that improvement?

_____

_____

_____

_____

** Rob recognized right away one blessing of cancer: it quickly drove him to his knees to ask for God's help. At the same time, though, cancer had Rob on his feet crying out, "This cancer is not bigger than God!" What rallying cry do you have—or might you adopt—for this battle your loved one is fighting?

_____

_____

2. When it came time to tell their kids about the cancer, Rob and Barbi chose this strategy: *Be honest with the children and invite them into the process*. Rob acknowledges that the severity of his cancer would have impacted the kind of conversation he and Barbi would have had with his sons.

   In what ways, if any, are you finding yourself in a support role not only for your loved one but also perhaps for that person's children, family members, or friends? What are you doing to take care of yourself so that you can keep giving?

Trusting God With Cancer

_____

_____

_____

_____

As exhausting as caregiving is, think about it for a moment as a privilege. What can you appreciate about this difficult journey you're traveling with someone you love?

_____

_____

_____

People die from cancer, and addressing death is rarely easy. Briefly describe your attitude toward death and how it is impacting—positively and/or negatively—your efforts to support your loved one. If your perspective on death is less than helpful, where will you turn for counsel and encouragement for yourself? If you would like to know more about death, take a look at page 93for resources.

_____

_____

_____

Lesson 4: Telling the Kids

3. After watching Rob in the pool with the boys, throwing them into the air and having them splash into the water again and again, Barbi dubbed this Raban approach to healing "the new face of cancer."

What can you do to encourage your loved one to give cancer a new face? Consider his/her passions and joys.

_____

_____

_____

For Rob, his physical activity and playing sports with his sons were signs of normalcy and, he noted, reassurance to the boys and to Rob himself that he was still alive. What activity, hobby, passion, or pastime can you help your loved one continue doing that might be a comforting sign of normalcy?

_____

_____

_____

If you are a follower of Jesus, walking alongside someone who has cancer is a chance to show that person, your family, and yourself the true meaning of faith. The diagnosis of cancer and its subsequent treatment are opportunities to demonstrate trusting your heavenly Father, praying, submitting to God's will, and asking for His help. As you walk alongside your loved one as he/she battles this evil disease, what sort of example will you be for him/her, for his/her children, perhaps for your own children, and for anyone else who is watching you?

_____

_____

_____

_____

The LORD is my light and my salvation; Whom shall I fear? The LORD is the strength of my life; Of whom shall I be afraid?

Psalm 27:1 NKJV

Lesson 5
Dreams That Matter

CANCER FIGHTERS

1. Experts say that everyone dreams. If that's the case, not everyone remembers their dreams—and not everyone who dreams and remembers them understands their dreams. Those gifted with good memories and remarkable insight can be encouraged by their dreams just as Rob was.

    Do you frequently remember your dreams? When, if ever, did a dream you remembered when you awoke have either a relevant message for you or a significant impact on you?

    _____

    _____

    The first dream Rob describes left him with a steely, lock-jawed determination to survive this cancer. His second dream served him as a source of comfort for a long time. What are your regular go-tos for inspiration in your fight against cancer? What are your regular go-tos for comfort? Which of these go-tos can you go to on

Trusting God With Cancer

your own? Which ones do you need help to go to? Let your caregiver know.

_____

_____

_____

_____

_____

2. Besides being a lasting source of comfort, Rob's second dream made a good point about the value of taking a break from big things like cancer and day-to-day things like homework.

What have you discovered that gives you a break from cancer? Or what would you like to try?

_____

_____

_____

** What, if anything, could your caregiver do to help you take a break from cancer? Let your caregiver know.

_____

_____

_____

Lesson 5: Dreams That Matter

3. Remember Rob's week of tests—of a bone marrow biopsy, a nuclear PET scan, a CT scan with contrast, a bone scan, an echocardiogram, and a spinal tap? Well, that was also the week of Rob's two dreams. Despite all the medical appointments and the big question mark about his diagnosis, Rob knew peace. In fact, he remembers knowing "the peace God gives that 'surpasses all understanding.'"

   Where do you go or what do you do when you need to experience some peace?

   _____

   When, if ever, have you felt that peace that "surpasses all understanding"? Why did you know it was from God?

   _____

   If you would like to know that kind of peace, simply ask God for that gift.

CAREGIVERS

1. Experts say that everyone dreams. If that's the case, not everyone remembers their dreams—and not everyone who dreams and remembers them understands their dreams. Those gifted with good memories and remarkable insight can be encouraged by their dreams just as Rob was.

   Do you frequently remember your dreams? When, if ever, did a dream you remembered when you awoke

Trusting God With Cancer

have either a relevant message for you or a significant impact on you?

_____

_____

The first dream Rob describes left him with a steely, lock-jawed determination to survive this cancer. His second dream long served him as a source of comfort. What are your regular go-tos for inspiration in your ongoing role as caregiver? What are your regular go-tos for comfort? Be sure to make time for them.

_____

_____

_____

_____

2. Besides being a lasting source of comfort, Rob's second dream made a good point about the value of taking a break from big things like cancer and day-to-day things like homework.

What have you discovered that gives you a break from thinking about cancer? Or what would you like to try?

_____

_____

Lesson 5: Dreams That Matter

** What might give your loved one a break from cancer? Be creative—and brainstorm with your loved one too.

_____

_____

_____

3. This was the week of tests for Rob—a bone marrow biopsy, a nuclear PET scan, a CT scan with contrast, a bone scan, an echocardiogram, and a spinal tap—but it was also the week of Rob's two dreams. Despite all the medical appointments and the big question mark about his diagnosis, Rob knew peace. In fact, he remembers knowing "the peace God gives that 'surpasses all understanding.'"

Where do you go or what do you do when you need to experience some peace?

_____

When, if ever, have you felt that peace that "surpasses all understanding"? Why did you know it was from God?

_____

If you would like to know that kind of peace, simply ask God for that gift.

You will keep him in perfect peace, Whose mind is stayed on You, Because he trusts in You.

Isaiah 26:3 NKJV

41

Lesson 6
A Week of Testing

CANCER FIGHTERS

1. Doctors use various tests to diagnose cancer, to determine its location, and to develop a treatment plan.

    Which of these tests that Rob had did you undergo? What, if anything, did you learn about his description of each?

    Echocardiogram

    _____

    Nuclear PET scan

    _____

    Abdominal/pelvic CT scan

    _____

    Spinal tap

    _____

Lesson 6: A Week of Testing

Bone marrow aspiration

_____

At what moment of the testing, if any, did you learn that you are much stronger than you probably give yourself credit for? Congratulate yourself for that!

_____

If you're still at odds with God over your cancer, please, please, please humble yourself and invite God into the situation. He wants to help you. Take a look at page 93 for resources.

2. In the Old Testament book of Job, the author describes Job as an upright man whom God loved. Yet we read that Job lost thousands of sheep, camels, and other livestock, many crops, his children, his position in the community, his possessions, and his physical health. No wonder he cried out to God—paraphrased—"What the heck did I do to deserve this, God?"

> ** Have you felt the kind of pain Job undoubtedly did? If so, what have you done with that pain, with any fear that accompanies your diagnosis, or with your anger that God would allow this to happen to you? Don't keep it inside. Talk to a friend, counselor, or pastor. Pray, write in a journal, scream, let yourself cry.

_____

_____

Trusting God With Cancer

_____

_____

_____

Near the end of the long book of Job, God spoke to this devoted man who had lost everything. On page 82, you can read some of what God said to Job. After that quote, Rob wrote, "God is simply, yet powerfully pointing out who Job isn't and who God is." Explain what you understand from this page in the book about "who Job isn't." What has Job realized about who he isn't? Be specific.

_____

_____

_____

_____

What do you learn from page 82 about who God is? What do your insights mean to you personally?

_____

_____

_____

_____

Lesson 6: A Week of Testing

3. Rob maintains that "Will God cure me?" is not the main issue in this battle against cancer. The main issue is *Will you crumble under your fear of cancer, will you tough it out on your own, or will you turn to the One who created you and choose to trust in Him?*

What, if anything, keeps you from choosing to trust God? Does He seem distant or uninterested? Have you had a bad experience in a church? Something else?

_____

_____

Cancer reminded Rob that he was not in control of the circumstances of his life or of what was going on with his body. Rob wrote, "Cancer reminded me of how truly weak I am, yet it gave me opportunity after opportunity to see how truly strong and good God is." What weaknesses have your diagnosis and battle against cancer revealed to you?

_____

_____

What opportunity—if any—have you taken to see how strong and how good God is? What specific event might you entrust to Him today?

_____

_____

Why does it make (at least a little) sense that choosing to trust God in His sovereignty, strength, power, and love would be key to winning the battle against cancer?

_____

_____

_____

CAREGIVERS

1. Doctors use various tests to diagnose cancer, to determine the extent of its spread, and to develop a treatment plan.

   Do you know/remember which of these tests your loved one had to undergo? What is at least one thing you learned about each from Rob's description?

   Echocardiogram

   _____

   Nuclear PET scan

   _____

   Abdominal/pelvic CT scan

   _____

   Spinal tap

   _____

Lesson 6: A Week of Testing

Bone marrow aspiration

———————————————

At what moment of the testing did you realize that your loved one was stronger than you thought—or stronger than even he/she thought? Affirm your loved one for the courage and strength you saw then and that you see now.

———————————————

If you're still at odds with God over your loved one's cancer, please, please, please humble yourself and invite God into the situation. He wants to help you. Take a look at page 93 for resources.

2. In the Old Testament book of Job, the author describes Job as an upright man whom God loved. Yet we read that Job lost thousands of sheep, camels, and other livestock, many crops, his children, his position in the community, his possessions, and his physical health. No wonder he cried out to God—paraphrased—"What the heck did I do to deserve this, God?"

> ** You may have felt the kind of pain Job undoubtedly did. If so, what did you do with that pain? What are you doing now with any fear that accompanies your loved one's diagnosis or with your anger that God would allow this to happen to someone you love? Don't keep it inside. Talk to a friend, counselor, or pastor. Pray, write in a journal, scream, let yourself cry.

Trusting God With Cancer

_____

_____

_____

_____

Near the end of the long book of Job, God speaks to this devoted man who had lost everything. On page 82, you can read some of what God said to Job. After that quote, Rob wrote, "God is simply, yet powerfully pointing out who Job isn't and who God is." Explain what you understand from this page in the book about "who Job isn't." What has Job realized about who he isn't? Be specific.

_____

_____

_____

_____

What do you learn from page 82 about who God is? What do your insights mean to you personally?

_____

_____

_____

Lesson 6: A Week of Testing

3. Rob maintains that "Will God cure me?" is not the main issue in this battle against cancer. The main issue is *Will you crumble under your fear of cancer, will you tough it out on your own, or will you turn to the One who created you and choose to trust in Him?*

What, if anything, keeps you from choosing to trust God? Does He seem distant or uninterested? Have you had a bad experience in a church? Something else?

_____

_____

_____

Cancer reminded Rob that he was not in control of the circumstances of his life or even what was going on with his body. Rob wrote, "Cancer reminded me of how truly weak I am, yet it gave me opportunity after opportunity to see how truly strong and good God is." What life experience reminded you of your weakness? Why can that reminder be a good thing?

_____

_____

_____

Think back over the recent past or even the distant past. What opportunity—if any—have you taken to see how strong and good God is? What specific event

Trusting God With Cancer

might you entrust to Him today?

_____

_____

Why does it make (at least a little) sense that choosing to trust God in His sovereignty, strength, power, and love would be key in supporting your loved one's battle against cancer? What positive effect might your choice to trust God have on your loved one?

_____

_____

_____

_____

> *I know that you can do all things, and that no purpose of yours can be thwarted.... Therefore I have uttered what I did not understand, things too wonderful for me, which I did not know.*
>
> Job responds to the Lord (Job 42:2-3)

Lesson 7
"Have a *Little* Faith"

CANCER FIGHTERS

1. Cancer. There are no guarantees about the outcome of the treatment. This evil disease is damn scary stuff. The fight requires faith—faith in your doctor, in medicine, in your ability to be strong, and/or in your God. Cancer is big, God is bigger, but your faith doesn't have to be big at all.

   > When he heard in his heart, "Rob, have a *little* faith," Rob thought right away of Jesus' reference to a mustard seed of faith (Matthew 17:20). A mustard seed is only 1 or 2 millimeters in diameter (0.039 to 0.079 inches). Rob decided he could have a *little* faith. Can you? Why or why not?

   _____

   _____

   If you would want to grow your faith, take a look at page 93 for resources. Whether you're a long-time follower of Jesus or just curious about Him, you'll find some suggestions.

Trusting God With Cancer

2. Simply put, prayer is having an open, honest conversation with God, and you can talk to Him any day of the week, anytime, anywhere, about anything. God loves you, He loves listening to you and talking to you, and He loves blessing you.

When you hear the word *prayer*, what comes to mind?

_____

What role is prayer playing—if any—in your battle against cancer? Why is prayer prominent, absent, or somewhere in between?

_____

_____

Realizing that God already knows our thoughts, Rob spoke to Him honestly about his fears. By not holding back, Rob learned that God can handle our honesty, our raw pain, our unfiltered rage, whatever we're feeling, thinking, and telling Him. Have you learned that lesson? If so, when—and how is that truth helping you now? If you haven't learned that God can handle anything you share with Him, why are you holding back? Telling God about the reason you're holding back would be a great starting point for an honest conversation with Him.

_____

_____

Lesson 7: "Have a Little Faith"

_____

_____

_____

3. We know all too well that God doesn't heal everyone. A person and all who love him might have prayed with faith and prayed faithfully, yet he/she died. Rob admits to not having a good answer for why God allows some people to live longer than others. But—Rob continues—God does call all of us to have faith in Him, to trust in the goodness of His plan, and to leave the outcome in His hands.

> ** Rob's dear friend Laura died of cancer despite praying and being prayed for. Before she passed, what perspective and hope helped her come to peace with God's plan for her? See pages 96-97 and/or 2 Corinthians 4:16-18 in a Bible. What hope does Laura's example offer you?

_____

_____

_____

What do you believe will happen to you after you die whether you die of cancer sooner or something else later? Explain why you hold that belief and why it is or isn't a source of comfort and strength. (If you want a better understanding of death and what comes after, turn to page 93 for resources.)

CAREGIVERS

1. Cancer. There are no guarantees about the outcome of the treatment. This evil disease is damn scary stuff. The fight requires faith—faith in doctors, in medicine, in the patient's ability to be strong, and/or in God. Cancer is big, God is bigger, but your faith doesn't have to be big at all.

   > When he heard in his heart, "Rob, have a *little* faith," Rob thought right away of Jesus' reference to a mustard seed of faith (Matthew 17:20). A mustard seed is only 1 or 2 millimeters in diameter (0.039 to 0.079 inches). Rob decided he could have a *little* faith. Can you? Why or why not?

   > _____

   > _____

   > If you would want to grow your faith, take a look at page 93 for resources. Whether you're a long-time follower of Jesus or just curious about Him, you'll find some suggestions.

1. Simply put, prayer is having an open, honest conversation with God, and you can talk to Him any day of the week, anytime, anywhere, about anything. God loves you, He loves listening to you and talking to you, and He loves blessing you.

   > When you hear the word *prayer*, what comes to mind?

   > _____

Lesson 7: "Have a Little Faith"

What role is prayer playing—if any—in your efforts to support your loved one? Why is prayer prominent, absent, or somewhere in between?

_____

_____

Realizing that God already knows our thoughts, Rob spoke to Him honestly about his fears. By not holding back, Rob learned that God can handle our honesty, our raw pain, our unfiltered rage, whatever we're feeling, thinking, and telling Him. Have you learned that lesson? If so, when—and how is that truth helping you now? If you haven't learned that God can handle anything you share with Him, why are you holding back? Telling God about the reason you're holding back would be a great starting point for an honest conversation with Him.

_____

_____

_____

_____

_____

2. We know all too well that God doesn't heal everyone. A person and all who love him might have prayed with faith and prayed faithfully, yet he/she died. Rob admits to not

having a good answer for why God allows some people to live longer than others. But—Rob continues—God does call all of us to have faith in Him, to trust in the goodness of His plan, and to leave the outcome in His hands.

> ** Rob's dear friend Laura died of cancer despite praying and being prayed for. Before she passed, what perspective and hope helped her come to peace with God's plan for her? See pages 96-97 and/or 2 Corinthians 4:16-18 in a Bible. What hope does Laura's example offer you?

_____

_____

_____

What do you believe will happen to you after you die? Explain why you hold that belief; why it is or isn't a source of comfort and strength; and how your belief might be impacting your loved one for good or not for good. (If you want an understanding of death and what comes after that will give you more hope, turn to page 93 for resources.)

May the God of hope fill you with all joy and peace in believing, so that by the power of the Holy Spirit you may abound in hope.

Romans 15:13 ESV

Lesson 8
Chemo: Embrace It!

CANCER FIGHTERS

1. Think about what you've seen of Rob's attitude and his actions… from titling this chapter to calling out "F… you, Satan!" to welcoming Karen and Barbi's company at chemo to enjoying Cindy's banter. Rob recognized that cancer is a crucible that, among other effects, clarifies what is really important. So Rob was all in to fight this cancer. He was fighting to be with his family, and that gave Rob purpose, motivation, and strength.

    What do you appreciate about Rob's approach to his fight against cancer? Be specific.

    _____
    _____
    _____
    _____

What attitude shift or specific action, if any, will you try out this week and perhaps adopt for yourself?

_____

_____

**What has the crucible of cancer taught you? What has it helped you understand about your priorities?

_____

_____

_____

2. You may have been surprised to read that, in Rob's experience, the chemotherapy room was "truly... one of the most life-affirming environments I've ever been in." He also commented on Cindy's banter that prompted some laughter and prevented self-pity.

What was/is your chemotherapy room like? What was/is its greatest strength?

_____

_____

Visualization was important in Rob's battle. Read aloud the long paragraph on page 116. What role has visualization played, if any, in your fight? Why has it been—or might it be—helpful?

Lesson 8: Chemo: Embrace It!

_____

_____

When talking about the negative side effects of chemo — nausea, hair loss, mouth sores, anal sores, stomach pain, neuropathy, bone pain/creaking, fatigue — Rob wrote, "But I learned that I can do hard, I can do unpleasant, and I can even do painful. And you can, too, especially when your life is on the line. Cancer will reveal marvelous strengths you never knew you had." If you can, give an example of when you were surprised by your strength. If you can't think of one, your caregiver might be able to help!

_____

_____

_____

3. Rob wrote, "Faith becomes real faith when we don't allow circumstances to sway us from what we know to be true about God."

Do you agree or disagree? Explain.

_____

_____

_____

Trusting God With Cancer

Cancer definitely brings with it circumstances that might challenge a person's faith in God. But God can handle our rage and even five F-bombs in a single sentence. Besides, He may allow pain in your life... for your benefit. (Remember Rob's amazing round of golf!) At this point of the battle, is your faith in God stronger or weaker? Why do you think that's the case?

_____

_____

_____

Rob suggests that the fatigue brought on by chemo can be time with God, an opportunity to learn from God, and—something we probably wouldn't volunteer for—a season of character growth and strengthening. If you're struggling with fatigue, are you open to using it to spend time with God? Why or why not?

_____

_____

What evidence of character growth have you noticed since your cancer diagnosis? Again, if you aren't sure, your caregiver might be able to help.

_____

_____

Lesson 8: Chemo: Embrace It!

CAREGIVERS

1. Think about what you've seen of Rob's attitude and his actions... from titling this chapter to calling out "F... you, Satan!" to welcoming Karen and Barbi's company at chemo to enjoying Cindy's banter. Rob recognized that cancer is a crucible that, among other effects, clarifies what is really important. So Rob was all in to fight this cancer. He was fighting to be with his family, and that gave Rob purpose, motivation, and strength.

   What encouragement do you find in Rob's attitude and actions as he fought cancer?

   _____

   _____

   _____

   _____

   As you read this chapter, what new way to support your loved one—if any—came to mind? When will you try it out?

   _____

   _____

   **In what way(s) is your loved one's fight against cancer a crucible for you? What lessons have you learned? What have you realized about your priorities?

Trusting God With Cancer

_____

_____

_____

_____

2. You may have been surprised to read that, in Rob's experience, the chemotherapy room was "truly... one of the most life-affirming environments I've ever been in." He also commented on Cindy's banter that prompted some laughter and prevented self-pity.

   Rob offers vivid descriptions of his experience with Cytoxin, Adiramycin, Vincristine, and Prednisone. What were the benefits of your reading about these challenges of the chemotherapy process?

   _____

   _____

   What did you learn about the side effects—nausea, hair loss, mouth sores, anal sores, stomach pain, neuropathy, bone pain/creaking, fatigue? What overriding impression did you take away from Rob's discussion of chemo?

   _____

   _____

   _____

Lesson 8: Chemo: Embrace It!

In what way, if any, might visualization help you in your role as caregiver? What "marvelous strength you never knew you had" is your caring for your loved one revealing? Be ready to tell your loved one what "marvelous strength" you have seen in him/her.

_____

_____

_____

3. Rob wrote, "Faith becomes real faith when we don't allow circumstances to sway us from what we know to be true about God."

   Do you agree or disagree? Explain.

_____

_____

_____

Cancer definitely brings with it circumstances that might challenge a CANCER FIGHTER'S or a CAREGIVER'S faith in God. After all, you didn't expect, plan, or choose this role of caregiver. You are undoubtedly dealing with the pain of seeing someone you love suffer, you might be exhausted, and you may be angry at God. But God can handle our rage and even five F-bombs in a single sentence. Besides, He may allow pain in your life... for your benefit. (Remember

Trusting God With Cancer

Rob's amazing round of golf!) At this point of the journey, is your faith in God stronger or weaker? Why do you think that's the case?

_____

_____

_____

What evidence of your own character growth have you noticed since your role as caregiver began? (Again, be ready to help your loved one recognize his/her own growth.)

_____

_____

_____

What has God been teaching you about life, Himself, and/or yourself?

_____

_____

_____

_____

Lesson 8: Chemo: Embrace It!

Bottom line, are you willing to acknowledge that some good is coming out of great pain? Identify some of the good you see—or explain why you think nothing good can come out of this pain.

_____

_____

_____

We rejoice in our sufferings, knowing that suffering produces endurance, and endurance produces character, character produces hope.

Romans 5:3-4 ESV

Lesson 9
Family, Friends, and the Internet

CANCER FIGHTERS

1. Rob was overwhelmed by the love, thoughtfulness, and support of people who knew him and his family and wanted to come alongside them in this battle. People brought home-cooked meals, one couple became the family's official—as in *consistent*—carpool drivers, the guys at work shaved their heads, and basketball buddies took Lefty all around the world…and sent ransom notes. Yet submitting to kindness was not easy for Rob, and it may not be easy for you.

    Read—and when you're in group, have someone read aloud—the first two paragraphs on page 131. What statements or phrases could have been your own words? Be specific.

    _____

    _____

Lesson 9: Family, Friends, and the Internet

_____

_____

_____

On a scale of 1 to 10, with 10 being very uncomfortable, how easy is it for you to submit to kindness? Is that an improvement over, say, a month ago? Why or why not?

_____

_____

What might you do to become more accepting of people's kindness and loving service? What truths can you remind yourself of and/or what simple self-talk might help?

_____

_____

_____

2. Google "cancer." In April 2020 over 900 million search results appeared. A Google search of "alternative cures for cancer" brought more than 13 million results. This access to information is great if you're interested—and if you have time to do the research and reading. Rob didn't: he had to fight. He also realized that he could no way master the body of knowledge about cancer that exists.

Trusting God With Cancer

Has Google been a friend or an enemy to you since your diagnosis? Explain.

_____

_____

_____

Likewise, has social media, including your email, been a friend or an enemy? Explain.

_____

_____

_____

Rob realized the importance of having a gatekeeper, and Barbi was a lifesaver in that regard. She freed up time and energy that Rob could invest in healing. Do you have a gatekeeper? If so, never hesitate to express your gratitude. If you don't have a gatekeeper, who might take on that role for you? Or where might you find a likely candidate?

_____

3. Self-care is more than just a trendy buzzword. Practicing self-care is essential to fighting the battle against cancer. Yet self-care often needs to be learned, and sometimes the way we think needs to be rewired. For Rob—and maybe for you—self-care seemed a self-centered way of living

Lesson 9: Family, Friends, and the Internet

that felt wrong and even shameful. As he wrote, "I needed to give myself permission to take care of myself and not see it as selfishness."

> ** Explain to yourself in your own words why self-care is critical for you in this battle.

_____

_____

_____

Healthy boundaries—both defined and enforced— are key to self-care. In what specific situations could your boundaries be stronger? What will you do to strengthen them?

_____

_____

_____

What are some specific things you can do that would qualify as self-care? Make a list and choose one to enjoy and/or work on this week.

_____

_____

_____

Trusting God With Cancer

CAREGIVERS

1. Rob was overwhelmed by the love, thoughtfulness, and support of people who knew him and his family and wanted to come alongside them in this battle. People brought home-cooked meals, one couple became the family's official—as in *consistent*—carpool drivers, the guys at work shaved their heads, and basketball buddies took Lefty all around the world...and sent ransom notes. Yet submitting to kindness was not easy for Rob, and it may not be easy for your loved one.

   If there have been sparks in your relationship with your loved one since you became a caregiver, what role might his/her reluctance and even inability to submit to kindness be playing in that conflict? Think about your loved one's upbringing, life, and personality.

   _____

   _____

   _____

   Read the first two paragraphs on page 131. What statements or phrases might express what your loved one is dealing with? (You might even ask!)

   _____

   _____

   _____

Lesson 9: Family, Friends, and the Internet

What impact might this insight have on your caregiving? Be specific.

_____

_____

_____

2. Google "cancer." In April 2020 over 900 million search results appeared. A Google search of "alternative cures for cancer" brought more than 13 million results. This access to information is great if you're interested—and if you have time to do the research and reading. Rob didn't: he had to fight. He also realized that he could no way master the body of knowledge about cancer that exists.

    Has Google been a friend or an enemy to you since your loved one's diagnosis? Explain.

    _____

    _____

    _____

    Likewise, has social media, including your email, been a friend or an enemy? Explain.

    _____

    _____

    _____

Trusting God With Cancer

Whatever your answers, the point is that information overload is a very real possibility. No wonder a person fighting cancer needs a gatekeeper! Is this an aspect of your role? If so, what are you doing? Could you be doing anything else as gatekeeper? If you aren't currently serving in this capacity, could you? What does your loved one need in terms of a gatekeeper? Write a job description for yourself and run it by your loved one.

_____

_____

_____

3. Self-care is more than just a trendy buzzword. Practicing self-care is essential to both fighting the battle against cancer and supporting the person who is in the fight. Yet self-care often needs to be learned, and sometimes the way we think needs to be rewired. For Rob—and maybe for you—self-care seemed a self-centered way of living that felt wrong and even shameful. As he wrote, "I needed to give myself permission to take care of myself and not see it as selfishness."

> ** Explain to yourself in your own words why self-care is critical for you as you take care of the loved one fighting cancer.

_____

_____

Lesson 9: Family, Friends, and the Internet

Healthy boundaries—both defined and enforced— are key to self-care. In what specific situations could your boundaries be stronger? What will you do to strengthen them?

What are some specific things you can do that would qualify as self-care? Make a list and choose one to enjoy and/or work on this week.

Trust in the Lord *with all your heart*
and lean not on your own understanding;
in all your ways submit to him,
and he will make your paths straight.

Proverbs 3:5-6

Lesson 10

Signs and Miracles

CANCER FIGHTERS

1. During Rob's cancer journey, he saw abundant evidence of God's presence with him. In fact, Rob says that God probably blessed him with more signs and miracles that he could recount or that he even recognized.

   > ** Read—and when in your group, read it aloud—the paragraph that begins on page 141 and continues on the next page. Rob's definition of miracles is broad because he includes what he calls "ordinary miracles." Which of those miracles have you experienced?

   _____

   _____

   _____

   Look back on your journey through the lens of Rob's definition of *miracles*. What miracles do you now see? What signs do you see that God was watching out for you, for instance, through the care and love of others?

Lesson 10: Signs and Miracles

———————————————————

———————————————————

2. Rob makes the comment that it takes a lot of faith to believe that a coincidence is merely a coincidence.

What do you make of Rob's nausea lifting as—he later learned—some Minnesota friends were praying for him?

———————————————————

———————————————————

What are your thoughts about both Barbi and Rob being awakened at 1:00 a.m. and learning that next morning that their son's teacher had been praying for them at 1:00 a.m.?

———————————————————

———————————————————

And when he was hospitalized with a fever, Rob was blessed with a great nurse who brought comfort and peace during the blood draw. But Rob learned the next morning that no 300-pound black male nurse was on staff at the hospital. Thoughts?

———————————————————

———————————————————

3. After sharing these examples, Rob made this simple statement: When you open up and pray to Jesus with "a *little* faith," you can expect miracles to happen.

> In chapter 7, Rob encouraged you to have "a *little* faith." What was your response, if any? Explain.
>
> _____
>
> _____
>
> _____
>
> Now Rob is encouraging you to pray with a *little* faith. What will you do, if anything, in response? Why?
>
> _____
>
> _____
>
> _____

CAREGIVERS

1. During Rob's cancer journey, he saw abundant evidence of God's presence with him. In fact, Rob says that God probably blessed him with more signs and miracles that he could recount or that he even recognized.

> ** Read—and when in your group, read aloud—the paragraph that begins on page 141 and continues on the next page. Rob's definition of miracles is broad because he includes what he calls "ordinary miracles."

Lesson 10: Signs and Miracles

> Which of those miracles have you experienced in your own life? Which have you seen unfold as you've journeyed with your loved one?

_____

_____

_____

Look back on your journey through the lens of Rob's definition of *miracles*. What miracles do you now see? What signs do you see that God was watching out for you, for instance, through the care and love of others?

_____

_____

_____

2. Rob makes the comment that it takes a lot of faith to believe that a coincidence is merely a coincidence.

   What do you make of Rob's nausea lifting as—he later learned—some Minnesota friends were praying for him?

   _____

   _____

   _____

What are your thoughts about both Barbi and Rob being awakened at 1:00 a.m. and learning that next morning that their son's teacher had been praying for them at 1:00 a.m.?

_____

_____

And when he was hospitalized with a fever, Rob was blessed with a great nurse who brought comfort and peace during the blood draw. But Rob learned the next morning that no 300-pound black male nurse was on staff at the hospital. Thoughts?

_____

_____

3. After sharing these examples, Rob made this simple statement: When you open up and pray to Jesus with "a *little* faith," you can expect miracles to happen.

In chapter 7, Rob encouraged you to have "a *little* faith." What was your response, if any? Explain.

_____

_____

_____

_____

Lesson 10: Signs and Miracles

Now Rob is encouraging you to pray with a *little* faith. What will you do, in anything, in response? Why?

_____

_____

_____

The Spirit helps us in our weakness. We do not know what we ought to pray for, but the Spirit himself intercedes for us through wordless groans....Christ Jesus who died—more than that, who was raised to life—is at the right hand of God and is also interceding for us.

Romans 8:26 and 34

Lesson 11

Strategies to Beat Cancer

When Rob was diagnosed with cancer, he didn't spend much time wondering how he got it. For him, the only thing that mattered when it came to cancer was how he was going to defeat it—and by God's grace, Rob did defeat it. Here Rob shares ten strategies that, in addition to God's grace, helped Rob win his fight against evil cancer.

Strategy #1: Trust God and give your cancer over to Him.

> Inviting God into the fight of your life is the single most important thing you can do to beat cancer. Even if you haven't had a relationship with God before, humble yourself and ask for His help. Openly share your fears with Him. Even tell Him you're not sure if He cares about you or if He even exists. Give your cancer over to God. Let Him fight the battle!

Strategy #2: Have a *little* faith, have a plan, and follow the plan.

> Don't complicate cancer. It's life-threatening, but that fact doesn't mean you can't beat it. You have cancer, and you want to get rid of it. God is bigger than cancer. Infinitely bigger. With a little faith and a doable plan and even a *little* belief, you will find that energy to follow that plan.

Lesson 11: Strategies to Beat Cancer

Strategy #3: Have a reason to live.

What if I die? you may be wondering, fearing. Rob asks, though, "Have you decided to live?" If so, what is your reason to live? If not, get to work finding a reason to live.

Strategy #4: Choose faith over reason.

Jumping into shark-infested water makes no sense (reason), but Jesus is calling you, "Follow Me!" As he thought about the fact that Jesus wasn't afraid to be in the water, Rob concluded He must be stronger than the cancer-sharks. Realizing he couldn't fight cancer alone, Rob knew he could fight with Jesus' strength and His presence with him in the battle (faith). Rob also concluded that the odds of survival are what you make them. The battle against cancer is not about being rational or even logical. The battle is about being faithful.

Strategy #5: Think positively!

Make the decision to live. Then make the decision that you will do anything you have to do in order to survive. Also, focus on positive thoughts of cure rather than any negative thoughts of loss. Know that the enemy will attack: Satan doesn't want you relying on God, knowing the Lord's peace, or standing strong as you do battle. Do whatever you need to do to think positively, stay positive, deny the negatives, and keep trusting God.

Strategy #6: Decide to be stronger at the end of chemo than at the beginning.

> Rob's goal of becoming physically stronger in the face of debilitating chemo inspired him to fight the evil disease. He encourages you to determine reasons for you yourself to set the same goal of getting physically stronger as the battle rages.

Strategy #7: Create visual anchors.

> During chemo—especially when Adriamycin was being administered—Rob pictured his bones made of pure marble: hard, solid, slippery, and not allowing any cancer to remain attached to them. He imagined a Pac-Man named Chemo eating up cancer cells. Choose visual anchors that will energize you to more fully embrace chemo.

Strategy #8: Keep working!

> As Dr. J told Rob, "You need to have a reason to get out of bed in the morning." When Rob's grandfather died, Rob found himself very busy taking over the family business as well as trying to save it in light of a 55% estate tax. Being this fully engaged in work helped him not be overly focused on his chemo. Work can do the same for you.

Lesson 11: Strategies to Beat Cancer

Strategy #9: Invite the kids into your healing.

If you have kids, let their watching eyes see you rely on God and then see how strong He enables you to be as you deal with adversity. Invite your kids into the healing process by giving them jobs around the house that you usually do. And let their love for you motivate you to dig deep for the courage and strength you need to press on. Stay involved in their lives—in their sports and schoolwork—and play hard with them.

Strategy #10: Have a gatekeeper.

Loved ones and concerned friends may struggle to find ways to best help you. You need these folks in your corner to support you as you fight cancer. But you don't need to ever be overwhelmed by well-meaning bits of advice on how best to treat your cancer. A gatekeeper can shield you as well as keep life going on the home, give you time for self-care, and ensure you have the energy you need to fight this all-important battle.

Trusting God With Cancer

CANCER FIGHTERS

Why are strategies important?

Which of these strategies are in place? Give a few examples of how those strategies are serving you well.

** Which strategies would you like to have in place that aren't in place right now? Choose one and determine the first step in establishing it.

Lesson 11: Strategies to Beat Cancer

CAREGIVERS

Why are strategies important?

_____

_____

Which of these strategies are in place? What, if anything, can you to do help your loved one strengthen those strategies?

_____

_____

_____

_____

** If you see some strategies that you would like to have in place for your loved one, talk together about that. Encourage your loved one to choose a strategy. Then, together determine how to best implement this strategy and the first step to take.

God is our refuge and strength,
an ever-present help in trouble.

Psalm 46:1

Epilogue

CANCER FIGHTERS

1. Rob experienced his battle against cancer as a season of profound spiritual growth.

   Read the second paragraph on page 175 and see some of the things Rob did to encourage his spiritual growth. Which one might you focus on this week? Be specific about what that will entail.

   _____

   _____

   _____

   In the third paragraph that begins on page 175, what one or two phrases or images do you find most helpful? Add them to your repertoire of visualizations if they aren't already there.

   _____

   _____

   _____

   _____

Trusting God With Cancer

2. "The blessing of cancer"?!? Yes! Throughout this book, Rob has shown us the blessings he experienced.

In what ways will you use for good the energy produced by your fear of cancer? Be specific.

_____

_____

_____

Why can acknowledging one's powerlessness be a good thing not just for Rob, but for you?

_____

_____

_____

Since being introduced to the concept in chapter 7, when—if at all—have you been able to "have a *little* faith"? What difference did that make in the circumstances you chose to have a *little* faith for? What difference did having that *little* faith make in you?

_____

_____

_____

_____

Epilogue

3. Gratitude can lighten life's burdens and generate hope.

Consider keeping a gratitude journal. Every day name at least one thing for which you are genuinely grateful. Once you get into practice—once you start looking for and seeing reasons to be grateful—you might up your daily minimum to two or three! Even if you don't write it down anywhere, identify one thing you are grateful for today.

_____

_____

** Right now you may be feeling grateful for Rob's book and the encouragement and wisdom he has offered. Share at least one valuable takeaway from your reading and your discussion of *Trusting God with Cancer*.

_____

_____

_____

Trusting God With Cancer

CAREGIVERS

1. Rob experienced his battle against cancer as a season of profound spiritual growth.

   Read the second paragraph on page 175 and see some of the things Rob did to encourage his spiritual growth. Some of those pertain more to your loved one, but not all. Which action might you focus on this week for your own spiritual growth? Be specific about what that will entail.

   _____

   _____

   _____

   In the third paragraph that begins on page 175, what one or two phrases or images do you find most helpful as you encourage and pray for your loved one? Add them to your repertoire of visualizations if they aren't already there.

   _____

   _____

   _____

   _____

Epilogue

2. "The blessing of cancer"?!? Yes! Throughout this book, Rob has shown us the blessings he experienced.

In what ways will you use for good the energy produced by your fear of cancer? Be specific.

_____

_____

_____

Why can acknowledging one's powerlessness be a good thing not just for Rob, but for you?

_____

_____

_____

Since being introduced to the concept in chapter 7, when—if at all—have you been able to "have a *little* faith"? What difference did that make in the circumstances you chose to have a *little* faith for? What difference did having that *little* faith make in you?

_____

_____

_____

_____

3. Gratitude can lighten life's burdens and generate hope.

Consider keeping a gratitude journal. Every day name at least one thing for which you are genuinely grateful. Once you get into practice—once you start looking for and seeing reasons to be grateful—you might up your daily minimum to two or three! Even if you don't write it down anywhere, identify one thing you are grateful for today.

** Right now you may be feeling grateful for Rob's book and the encouragement and wisdom he has offered. Share at least one valuable takeaway from your reading and your discussion of *Trusting God with Cancer*.

Resources

The First Step: An Invitation

When I put my faith in Jesus, I gave up my claim on my life. Maybe my coming to this point looks to some people like I was giving up and giving in, but quite the opposite is true. The choice to surrender one's life—one's self—to Jesus is a conscious step necessary for dropping a false belief ("I am sovereign") and for claiming a truth ("God is sovereign").

I need Jesus. You need Jesus. Surrender yourself to Him. Submit your own plans for your life to Him. And be saved. Choose—as I did—to have faith in Him, faith that His death on the cross covered the cost of my sin and yours. Choose—as I did—to trust that the almighty Creator of the universe has not only the *power* to save you, but also the *desire* to save you.

Acknowledge to God the ways you fall short of your own standards for yourself. Then confess to God the ways you fall far short of His standards for you, the ways you have sinned. Ask God for His forgiveness... receive it... and tell Jesus that you want to live with Him as your Savior and Lord. With that decision and prayer, you have been adopted as God's son/daughter and entered the family of God. Know that your heavenly Father loves to bless His children with His peace and comfort, a new freedom and strength, a sense of purpose and belonging, wisdom and guidance, and so much more!

A Handful of Foundational Truths

God so loved the world, that he gave his only Son, that whoever believes in him shall not perish but have eternal life. — John 3:16

If we confess our sins, he is faithful and just to forgive us our sins and to cleanse us from all unrighteousness. — 1 John 1:9

If you confess with your mouth that Jesus is Lord and believe in your heart that God raised him from the dead, you will be saved. — Romans 10:9

God shows his love for us in that while we were still sinners, Christ died for us. — Romans 5:8

When we were dead in our transgressions, [God] made us alive together with Christ (by grace you have been saved). — Ephesians 2:5 NASB

Finding Answers to Questions

Below you'll find resources for questions that may have arisen as you read through and discussed the chapters. Know that GotQuestions is a great online resource (gotquestions.org). As its website says, "Your questions. Biblical answers" — and that organization has answered 607,384 Bible questions about God, Jesus, theology, and the Bible itself. You'll be able to find answers to many questions that arise as you read *Trusting God with Cancer*.

Resources

Resources for Specific Topics*

- Chapter #2: Why do bad things happen?

    o https://www.christianity.com/wiki/christian-life/why-do-bad-things-happen-to-good-people.html

    o Greg Laurie https://harvest.org/resources/devotion/why-do-bad-things-happen-to-good-people-2/

    o http://www.cruhighschool.com/resource/why-does-god-let-bad-things-happen/

- Chapter #3: What is a Christian supposed to do with anger, especially anger at God?

    o "Angry or Mad at God? Here's What's to Do" https://www.thehopeline.com/mad-at-god-2/

    o https://www.crosswalk.com/faith/spiritual-life/how-should-christians-deal-with-anger.html

    o https://www.focusonthefamily.com/get-help/when-your-anger-gets-the-best-of-you/

- Chapter #4: What happens when we die?

    o https://www.cru.org/us/en/how-to-know-god/what-happens-when-i-die.html

    o https://www.desiringgod.org/articles/what-happens-at-death

    o https://www.ligonier.org/learn/qas/when-person-dies-where-does-his-or-her-spirit-and/

- Chapter #6: What do I do to invite God into every situation of my life and walk with Him?

  o https://billygraham.org/answer/walk-with-god/

  o https://blog.lifeway.com/leadingmen/2019/04/23/10-ways-to-practically-improve-your-walk-with-christ/

  o https://www.crosswalk.com/faith/women/4-things-you-need-to-walk-with-god-daily.html

- Chapter #7: What do I do to grow my faith?

  o https://billygraham.org/story/9-ways-to-grow-in-your-faith/

  o https://www.whatchristianswanttoknow.com/how-to-increase-your-faith/

  o https://lifehopeandtruth.com/change/faith/how-to-grow-in-faith/

**If these website addresses (April 2020) are no longer current, googling the question being asked will yield many responses. Not all will be biblical. If you aren't sure about a source, don't hesitate to ask your group leader, a Christian friend, or a pastor for guidance before proceeding further.

Resources

Ideas for Leaders: Opening Each Group Time

Chapter #1 *Misdisagnosing a Sneeze*

It's so hard to forgive….

Corrie ten Boom Forgives https://justbetweenus. org/faith/inspirational-stories/christian-stories-of-forgiveness/

Chapter #2 *"Your Cancer Is Doubling on the Hour"*

Why do bad things happen?

Joni Eareckson Tada https://www.ligonier.org/learn/articles/turning-evil-its-head/

Chapter #3 *Finding New Hope*

I want to learn more about God.

"How Can I Get to Know God Better?" at gotquestions. org

"Understanding God" at https://www.allaboutgod. com/understanding-god.htm

Chapter #4 *Telling the Kids*

Do you have a battle cry?

The 101st Airborne Division: See "Currahee!" near the end of the article at https://www.artofmanliness.com/articles/battle-cries/

Chapter #5 *Dreams That Matter*

I want to know more about that peace that passes understanding.

Horatio Gates Spafford, writer of "It Is Well with My Soul," at https://www.christianpost.com/voices/the-peace-of-god-passes-all-understanding.html

Chapter #6 *A Week of Testing*

Rob advises, "If you are at odds with God, invite Him into the situation."

"Pastor John's Story: A Modern-Day Job" at https://vom.com.au/pastor-johns-story-a-modern-day-job/

Chapter #7 *"Have a Little Faith"*

Do heaven and hell exist?

Cru's Core Christian Beliefs: "Heaven and Hell" https://www.cru.org/us/en/train-and-grow/spiritual-growth/core-christian-beliefs/heaven-and-hell.html

"Jim Woodford's Testimony of Coming Back After Seeing Heaven and Hell" at https://www.godupdates.com/jim-woodford-testimony-seeing-heaven-hell/

Chapter #8 *Chemo: Embrace It!*

The fires of life's trials—cancer, chemo—are not for naught.

"Life's Trials: God's Refining Fire" (see especially Stages V-VI) at https://www.hopefortheheart.org/july-2013-letter-from-june-on-trials/

Resources

Chapter #9 *Family, Friends, and the Internet*

I want to be there for my friend, but I don't know what to say....

"5 Ways to Comfort People" at https://www.guideposts.org/friends-and-family/friends/5-ways-to-comfort-people

Chapter #10 *Signs and Miracles*

I want to see God at work in my life.

"Seeing God, Recognizing Him" (see the end of "Seeing God at Work in the Little Things") at https://www.patheos.com/blogs/kpyohannan/2018/09/seeing-god-work-little-things/

Chapter #11 *Strategies to Beat Cancer*

Benjamin Franklin wisely observed, "If you fail to plan, you are planning to fail." Here are six stories of great battle strategies. Choose one or two to share.

https://www.mentalfloss.com/article/50799/ruse-war-6-sneaky-brilliant-strategies